TABLE OF CONTENTS

INTRODUCTION

There are moments in life when we need reassurance, clarity, and control especially when the unexpected happens. Whether a condom broke, contraception was missed, or the timing just wasn't right, knowing that you have a safe, effective backup option matters. That's where emergency contraceptive pills come in.

This guide is designed to walk you through everything you need to know about using Levonorgestrel 1.5 mg emergency contraceptive tablets confidently and responsibly. It's not just about the science it's about your peace of mind, your health, and your right to make informed decisions about your body.

Inside, you'll find clear answers, helpful tips, and reassuring facts all written to support you through what can feel like an overwhelming

EMERGENCY CONTRACEPTIVE PILL ULTIMATE USAGE GUIDE (1.5mg LEVONORGESTREL)

Your Essential Step-by-Step Handbook for Safe, Timely, and Confident Use to Prevent Unplanned Pregnancy

RN Anita Jabs Surez

situation. No jargon. No fear. Just facts, compassion, and guidance.

You are not alone and you're in control.

CHAPTER 2: UNDERSTANDING EMERGENCY CONTRACEPTIVE PILLS

Emergency contraceptive pills (ECPs), often referred to as "the morning-after pill," are a safe and effective backup method of preventing pregnancy after unprotected sex or contraceptive failure (e.g., condom breakage or missed birth control pills).

What Are Emergency Contraceptive Pills?
ECPs contain hormones or hormone-like ingredients that prevent or delay ovulation, meaning they stop the release of an egg from the ovaries. Without an egg to meet sperm, pregnancy cannot occur. The most commonly used emergency contraceptive is Levonorgestrel (1.5 mg), a progestin hormone found in many daily birth control pills—but at a higher, one-time dose.

How Are They Different From Regular Birth Control?

While daily birth control is designed for ongoing prevention, ECPs are intended for occasional emergency use only. They are not meant to replace regular contraceptives but to serve as a second chance option when your primary method fails or isn't used.

Myths vs Facts

- Myth: ECPs cause abortion

  Fact: They do not end an existing pregnancy. They work before fertilization.
- Myth: You can't take ECPs more than once

  Fact: While not meant for regular use, they can be safely used more than once when needed.
- Myth: ECPs make you infertile

  Fact: There's no evidence they harm future fertility.

Types of Emergency Contraceptive Pills
- Levonorgestrel-based (like this product): Available without a prescription in many countries, including the UK.
- Ulipristal acetate (EllaOne®): Prescription-only in some regions, and may work slightly longer.

Who Can Use ECPs?
Emergency contraception is safe for most women, including teenagers and those who cannot use other hormonal methods. There are no age or weight limits that disqualifies its use, though efficacy may slightly reduce in women with higher body weight.

CHAPTER 3:

WHEN TO USE THIS PRODUCT

Emergency contraceptive pills (ECPs) are designed for specific situations when your regular birth control fails or isn't used. Knowing when to take an ECP like the 1.5 mg Levonorgestrel pill is essential for maximizing effectiveness and avoiding unintended pregnancy.

Situations When Emergency Contraception Is Recommended
Use this product if:
- You had unprotected sex (no contraception used).
- Your condom broke, slipped, or leaked during intercourse.
- You missed two or more active birth control pills in a row.
- Your contraceptive patch or ring became loose or detached.

- You were late getting a birth control injection (like Depo-Provera).
- You were forced into sex without protection (non-consensual encounter).
- You incorrectly used your fertility awareness method.
- You forgot or incorrectly used another form of birth control (like a diaphragm, cervical cap, or withdrawal).

The 72-Hour Window (3 Days)
This pill is most effective when taken as soon as possible, ideally within 12 to 24 hours after unprotected sex.
- Within 24 hours: Highest effectiveness (up to 95%)– 24 to 48 hours: Effectiveness drops slightly
- 48 to 72 hours: Still effective, but less so

After 72 hours, Levonorgestrel-based pills are not recommended, and you may need a different emergency option like ulipristal acetate or a copper IUD (consult a healthcare provider).

What If You're Unsure?

If you're not sure whether your contraception failed, or you're second-guessing the risk, it's better to be cautious. Emergency contraception is safe to use even if you later find out it wasn't needed.

Not for Ongoing Use

This product is not intended for routine birth control. It's a backup method not a replacement for consistent contraception.

CHAPTER 4:

HOW IT WORKS

The emergency contraceptive pill (ECP) in this guide contains 1.5 mg of Levonorgestrel, a synthetic hormone that helps prevent pregnancy after unprotected sex or contraceptive failure. Understanding how it works can give you peace of mind and help ensure it's used effectively.

What Is Levonorgestrel?
Levonorgestrel is a progestin, a hormone commonly used in many types of birth control pills. In emergency contraception, it's given in a higher, single dose to quickly interrupt the process of conception.

Mechanism of Action

Levonorgestrel prevents pregnancy in three key ways:

1. Delays or Inhibits Ovulation
   - The pill can prevent the release of an egg from the ovary, which means there's no egg for sperm to fertilize.
   - This is the primary way Levonorgestrel works when taken before ovulation.

2. Thickens Cervical Mucus
   - Makes it harder for sperm to travel through the cervix and reach the egg.

3. Alters the Uterine Lining
   - If ovulation has already occurred, the pill may make it more difficult for a fertilized egg to implant in the uterus.

Important to note:
- It does not terminate an existing pregnancy.
- It is not effective if implantation has already occurred.
- It will not protect against future unprotected sex during your cycle.

Time–Sensitive Action
The sooner you take the pill after unprotected intercourse, the better it works. Taking it within 12 hours offers the best chance of success.

CHAPTER 5:

RECOMMENDED USAGE GUIDELINES

Using emergency contraception effectively means understanding exactly when and how to take it for maximum protection. The guidelines below are designed to help you make informed, confident decisions when the unexpected happens.

When to Take the Pill
- As Soon As Possible:
  The emergency contraceptive pill works best when taken within 12 to 24 hours after unprotected sex.
  - Effectiveness:
    - Within 24 hours: up to 95% effective
    - Within 72 hours: around 85% effective
    - Up to 120 hours (5 days): May still work, but with reduced effectiveness.

Dosage Instructions
- Take one tablet (1.5 mg of Levonorgestrel) orally, with water.
- It can be taken with or without food, but eating something before can help reduce the chance of nausea.
- Do not take more than one dose unless advised by a medical professional.

If You Vomit
- If you vomit within 2 hours of taking the pill, it may not have been absorbed properly.
  - In this case, take another dose as soon as possible.
  - If vomiting persists, speak with a pharmacist or doctor for alternative options.

What If You Missed the 72-Hour Window?
- The effectiveness decreases, but some protection may still be possible up to 120 hours.
- However, seek medical advice immediately if you're outside the recommended window.

Important Reminders

- One-time use per incident: Each dose covers one unprotected sex event. If you have unprotected sex again, you'll need another dose.

- Not for regular use: This is for emergencies only, not as a substitute for daily birth control.

CHAPTER 6:

WHAT TO EXPECT AFTER TAKING IT

Taking an emergency contraceptive pill (ECP) like Levonorgestrel is a responsible step, and knowing what to expect afterward can ease anxiety and help you monitor your body appropriately.

1. Changes in Your Menstrual Cycle
- Period Timing: Your period may come earlier or later than usual, typically within 7 days of your expected date.
- Flow Differences: It might be heavier, lighter, or more spotty than normal. This is due to hormonal shifts from the pill.
- If your period is more than 7 days late, take a pregnancy test.

2. Common Side Effects (Short-Term)
These are typically mild and go away in a day or two:
- Nausea or upset stomach
- Headache
- Breast tenderness
- Dizziness or fatigue
- Mild abdominal pain or cramping
- Light spotting or breakthrough bleeding

These are signs your body is adjusting to the hormone. If they persist beyond 48 hours or become severe, consult a healthcare professional.

3. Signs the Pill Worked
There is no immediate "confirmation" the pill worked, but if you get your next period and it's fairly normal, it's a strong indicator. If you miss your period or it's unusually light, take a pregnancy test 3 weeks after use.

4. When to Seek Medical Advice
Contact a doctor or pharmacist if:
- Vomiting occurs within 2 hours of taking the pill

- You feel unusually unwell or develop severe lower abdominal pain (this could signal an ectopic pregnancy)
- Your period is more than 7 days late

5. Emotional Responses
It's normal to feel anxious, guilty, or overwhelmed after taking emergency contraception. Remember:
- You made a safe, responsible choice
- Support is available don't hesitate to speak with a trusted friend, counselor, or health provider

CHAPTER 7:

IMPORTANT SAFETY CONSIDERATIONS

While emergency contraceptive pills (ECPs) like Levonorgestrel are considered safe and effective for most women, it's essential to understand how to use them responsibly and when caution is necessary. Your safety always comes first.

1. Not for Regular Birth Control
- ECPs are not meant for routine contraception. They are designed for occasional, emergency use only.
- Frequent use can disrupt your menstrual cycle and is less effective than regular birth control methods like the pill, IUD, or implants.

2. Don't Exceed the Recommended Dose
- Only one 1.5mg tablet should be taken per emergency event.
- Taking more than one dose in a single 24-hour period won't increase effectiveness—it may instead lead to hormonal imbalance and side effects.

3. Timing Matters
- The sooner you take it, the better. Levonorgestrel is most effective within 72 hours (3 days) after unprotected sex.
- Effectiveness decreases each day—don't delay.

4. Age and Weight Factors
- It is approved for use by women of reproductive age, but consult a doctor if under 16.
- Effectiveness may be reduced in women over a certain weight or BMI (usually above 75kg or BMI >26). In these cases, consider discussing alternatives with a pharmacist or doctor.

5. Medication Interactions

Certain medications or supplements can reduce the effectiveness of emergency contraception, such as:
- Some epilepsy treatments (e.g., phenytoin, carbamazepine)
- HIV medications
- St. John's Wort
- Certain antibiotics

Always inform your doctor or pharmacist of any medications you are taking.

6. Not Protective Against STIs

Emergency contraceptive pills do not protect against sexually transmitted infections (STIs). If you believe you've been exposed, visit a clinic for testing and advice.

7. Pre-existing Health Conditions
While most women can safely take ECPs, speak with a healthcare provider if you:
- Have liver disease
- Are on long-term medications
- Have any history of hormonal disorders

8. Don't Use If Already Pregnant
Levonorgestrel will not terminate an existing pregnancy and should not be used as an abortion method.

Understanding these safety guidelines ensures you make empowered, informed decisions about your reproductive health. Always prioritize your well-being and don't hesitate to reach out to a medical professional if unsure.

CHAPTER 8:

POTENTIAL REACTIONS AND SIDE EFFECTS

Emergency contraceptive pills like Levonorgestrel are generally safe and well-tolerated. However, like all medications, they may cause temporary side effects in some women. Being aware of what to expect can help ease anxiety and support recovery.

1. Common Side Effects (Usually Mild & Short-Term)
These may appear within a few hours to a couple of days after taking the pill:

- Nausea or vomiting
- Headache
- Fatigue or dizziness
- Breast tenderness
- Lower abdominal pain or cramping

– Changes in your next period (earlier, later, heavier, or lighter than usual)

Tip: Taking the pill with food may reduce the chance of nausea.

2. Menstrual Irregularities
It's common for your next period to be:

– A few days early or late
– Lighter or heavier than usual
– Accompanied by spotting or breakthrough bleeding

If your period is more than 7 days late, or significantly different, take a pregnancy test.

3. Vomiting Shortly After Taking the Pill
– If you vomit within 2 hours of taking the pill, it may not have been absorbed.

- You should take another dose as soon as possible and speak to a pharmacist or healthcare provider.

4. Allergic Reactions (Rare)
Very rarely, someone may experience a mild allergic reaction such as:

- Rash or itching
- Swelling (especially of the face or throat)
- Difficulty breathing

If any of these symptoms occur, seek immediate medical attention.

5. Emotional Reactions
Some women report feeling:

- Anxious
- Irritable
- Low mood or emotional sensitivity

These symptoms usually resolve on their own within a few days. If they persist, speak to a healthcare provider.

6. Long-Term or Serious Side Effects
Levonorgestrel has been studied extensively and is not linked to long-term health issues when used occasionally and as directed. It does not affect future fertility, nor does it cause miscarriage.

⚠ When to See a Doctor
You should seek medical advice if you experience:

- Severe abdominal pain (could signal ectopic pregnancy)
- Heavy or prolonged bleeding
- Missed period after 3 weeks
- Persistent vomiting or headaches
- Signs of pregnancy despite taking the pill

—Most side effects are a temporary response to hormonal changes and not a cause for concern. With proper use and awareness, emergency contraception remains a safe, effective, and empowering option for preventing unintended pregnancy.

CHAPTER 9:

COMMON QUESTIONS ANSWERED (FAQs)

When it comes to emergency contraception, many women have similar concerns. This chapter addresses the most frequently asked questions to help you feel more informed, confident, and in control.

1. How effective is the emergency contraceptive pill?

When taken within 72 hours (3 days) of unprotected sex, Levonorgestrel is about 85–95% effective. The sooner it's taken, the better the chance of preventing pregnancy.

2. Can I take it more than once?
Yes, you can use it more than once, but it's not recommended as a regular method of contraception. Frequent use may cause irregular periods.

3. Does it protect me for the rest of the month?
No. It only works for the specific instance of unprotected sex. If you have unprotected sex again, you may need another dose or a long-term birth control method.

4. Will it affect my fertility?
No. There is no evidence that using emergency contraception affects your long-term ability to get pregnant.

5. What if I vomit after taking it?
If vomiting occurs within 2 hours, the pill may not be absorbed. You may need to take another dose.

6. Will it stop my period?
No. It might change the timing of your next period (earlier, later, lighter, or heavier), but it won't cancel it.

7. Can I use it during breastfeeding?
Yes. Levonorgestrel is safe during breastfeeding. A small amount may pass into breast milk, but it's not harmful to your baby.

8. What if I'm already pregnant?
Emergency contraception won't work if you're already pregnant, and it will not harm an existing pregnancy.

9. Can I take it while on birth control pills?
Yes. But if you missed regular pills or had a contraceptive failure, the emergency pill adds backup protection. Continue your regular birth control afterward.

10. Is it safe for teens and young adults?
Yes. It's approved and safe for women of reproductive age, including teenagers.

11. Can I drink alcohol after taking it?
Alcohol doesn't reduce the pill's effectiveness, but avoid excessive drinking to ensure you don't vomit or forget a follow-up.

12. Can I buy it without a prescription?
In the UK and many countries, yes. Emergency contraceptive pills are available over the counter at pharmacies.

13. What if I have a medical condition?Most women can use Levonorgestrel safely, but consult a healthcare provider if you have a chronic condition or are taking other medications.

14. Will it protect me from STIs?
No. Emergency contraception does not protect against sexually transmitted infections (STIs). Use condoms to reduce STI risk.

15. How can I avoid needing emergency contraception again?
Consider a reliable ongoing birth control method and always use condoms. Keep a pill on hand for true emergencies only.

CHAPTER 10: RESPONSIBLE AND INFORMED USE

Using emergency contraception wisely is not just about preventing pregnancy it's about understanding your body, making informed choices, and respecting your health. This chapter offers practical guidance on how to use the emergency contraceptive pill in a safe, responsible, and thoughtful way.

1. Use It for True Emergencies
Emergency contraception is designed for unexpected situations such as:
- Missed or broken condoms
- Missed birth control pills
- Unprotected sex
- Sexual assault

It is not intended as a regular form of contraception.

2. Know When to Take It
Timing is everything:
- For best results, take it within 24 hours.
- It can work up to 72 hours after unprotected sex but is less effective over time.

3. Keep One in Your Emergency Kit
Life happens. Having a pill available at home, especially if you're sexually active, can reduce stress and delay in moments of panic.

4. Be Honest With Yourself
Ask:
- Why do I need this pill today?
- Could I avoid this in the future with a better routine or protection plan?

Being responsible is also about learning from the moment.

5. Understand Its LimitationsIt does not:
- Protect against STIs
- Prevent pregnancy if you're already pregnant
- Replace the need for long-term birth control

It's a backup, not a main method.

6. Talk to a Healthcare Professional
Whether it's your first time using the pill or you have recurring situations, consider speaking with:
- A GP
- A nurse at a sexual health clinic
- A pharmacist

You deserve to make decisions based on trusted guidance.

7. Prioritise Long-Term Contraception
Emergency contraception shouldn't be your Plan A. If you're sexually active, explore options like:
- Birth control pills
- IUDs
- Implants
- Condoms (for STI protection too)

8. Practice Self-Care
Taking emergency contraception can bring up emotions relief, stress, guilt, or confusion. That's okay. Be kind to yourself. Stay hydrated, eat well, rest, and talk to someone if needed.

9. Stay Informed
Make it a habit to:
- Read trusted sources
- Learn about your cycle
- Track your periods
- Know your emergency options

Being informed helps you feel more in control and less anxious in the future.

10. Respect Your Body & BoundariesYou deserve respect in your choices, your relationships, and your health decisions. Using emergency contraception is your right, and doing so responsibly shows strength, not weakness.

Informed use is empowered use. The more you know, the more confident and in control you becomeabout your body, your choices, and your future.

CHAPTER 11:

HANDLING, STORAGE, AND EXPIRY

Proper storage and handling of your emergency contraceptive pill are just as important as using it correctly. This chapter will guide you on how to keep the medication safe, effective, and ready when needed.

1. Keep It in a Cool, Dry Place
Store your emergency contraceptive pill at room temperature, ideally between 15°C and 25°C (59°F–77°F). Avoid humid places like:
- Bathrooms
- Near windows or radiators
- Inside a hot car or gym bag

Moisture and heat can damage the pill and reduce its effectiveness.

2. Store in Original Packaging

Always keep the pill in its original blister pack or container until you're ready to use it. This:
- Protects it from light and moisture
- Keeps it properly labeled
- Ensures you can easily access the expiry date and instructions

3. Keep Out of Reach of Children

While emergency contraception is not harmful if accidentally consumed by others, it should always be kept out of reach of:
- Children
- Pets

Safe, private storage prevents misuse or confusion.

4. Don't Use Past Expiry

Check the expiry date before use. Expired emergency contraceptive pills:
- May lose potency
- Might not work as expected
- Could lead to failed contraception

It's a good idea to check the date every few months if you keep one in your personal emergency kit.

5. Traveling? Store It Smart

If you travel frequently:
- Keep the pill in your carry-on, not checked luggage (temperature may vary in cargo)
- Use a small container or pouch to prevent it from getting crushed or bent
- Keep it discreet but easily accessible

6. What If It Gets Damaged?

If the packaging is:
- Torn

– Crushed
– Exposed to water or heat

It's best not to use it. Purchase a replacement from a licensed pharmacy.

7. Dispose of Properly
If you need to dispose of an expired or damaged pill:
– Do not flush it down the toilet or throw it in the bin directly
– Follow local pharmacy disposal guidelines or return it to a pharmacy for safe disposal

By handling and storing your emergency contraception properly, you protect its effectiveness and ensure you're ready when you truly need it.

CHAPTER 13:

CONCLUSION

Emergency contraceptive pills serve as an important option for preventing unintended pregnancy when used correctly and responsibly. As you've learned throughout this guide, understanding how these pills work, when and how to use them, and the necessary precautions can empower you to make informed choices about your reproductive health.

Key Takeaways
- Emergency contraception is a safe and effective backup method, not a replacement for regular contraception.
- Timing is critical: the sooner you take the pill after unprotected intercourse, the better your chances of preventing pregnancy.

- Understanding potential side effects helps you prepare and avoid unnecessary worry.
- Always follow usage instructions carefully and keep the medication stored properly to maintain its effectiveness.
- Consult a healthcare professional if you have any doubts, experience severe side effects, or need advice on ongoing contraception.

Your Health, Your Choice. This guide is designed to help you feel confident and informed. Remember, your reproductive health is your personal journey. Whether you use emergency contraception once or as a part of your reproductive plan, making responsible choices is vital for your well-being.

Empowerment Through Knowledge
Having access to accurate information and understanding how to use emergency contraception correctly can reduce anxiety and help you take control of unexpected situations.

This book aims to be a trusted resource to help you feel prepared, safe, and supported.

Looking Ahead

Emergency contraceptive pills are just one tool in the broader spectrum of reproductive health options. Consider speaking with healthcare providers about long-term contraception methods to find what best fits your lifestyle and needs.

Thank you for choosing this guide as your resource. Your health matters, and being informed is the first step toward peace of mind and empowerment. Let us know how this has helped your journey. Yippee!!!

Printed in Dunstable, United Kingdom

71978079R00030